Bea's diabetes:

A parent's journey

By

Lucie Quest

Disclaimer

This book is not intended to be a substitute for the medical advice of a licensed physician. The reader should consult with their doctor in any matters relating to their child's health. Any advice and recommendations in this book are the author's personal thoughts and based on the author's own experiences. They are not intended to be a definitive set of instructions or medical advice. The author recognises that for any people mentioned in the book, their memories of the events described may be different from the authors own.

Contents

Introduction   3

Diagnosis   3

    How did I know Beatrice had Type 1 diabetes?   3

    How did I feel?   3

    What happened next?   4

Common comments made by others   5

Coping with Type 1 diabetes as a toddler   6

    The relentless hospital visits   6

    A toddlers interpretation of emotion   7

    How type 1 diabetes affects behaviour   8

How type 1 diabetes can impact your family   9

The practicalities   11

Micro-managing – the pressure to get it right (all the time)   13

Bed wetting   15

Dealing with hypos   16

Being ill with type 1 diabetes   18

Moving from injections to the pump   19

Pump Adjustments   26

School, child-minding and babysitting   28

    Uniform   30

    PE   31

Carbohydrate counting and eating out   32

    Calculating carbohydrates   33

    'Diabetic' chocolate and sweets   34

Travelling with type 1diabetes   35

Monetary support   37

The next steps   37

Acknowledgements   39

Introduction

I'm a mum to my son Wilfred, aged 4, and my daughter Beatrice, aged 6, who was diagnosed with type 1 diabetes at 2 years old. It was a very difficult time of adjustment for the whole family.

This book is aimed at others who care for a child with type 1 diabetes. It is not a scientific fact file; it is an honest account of living life with someone with type 1 diabetes. I have used my experience to provide some useful tips to help guide you through this steep learning curve, addressing the affects it has on the whole family and sharing some of my thoughts and feelings throughout Beatrice's first 4 years since diagnosis.

Diagnosis

How did I know Beatrice had Type 1 diabetes?

This always fills me with guilt. The bottom line is that we didn't know. She complained about walking, so we encouraged her to walk more often to get used it. She said she was tired, so we put her to bed earlier. She kept drinking loads in the evening and then would wet the bed, so we gave her less to drink at night. As far as we were concerned our little girl was going through the 'terrible two's.' It was only when she came downstairs for breakfast with blue lips one morning that I was concerned. My husband took her to the doctors in the morning and I got the phone call at work to say she was being taken to the hospital immediately. Her blood sugar level was so high that it couldn't be read by the blood glucose meter.

How did I feel?

I remember being in a room with doctors and nurses telling me that my 2 year old daughter had type 1 diabetes and me saying "Ok, so what do we do? Will it take very long as we really need to get home as my 8 month old son needs feeding" The reply was "Beatrice will be in hospital for at least a few days. One of you will need to stay here". I genuinely thought she was joking until I realised I was the only one smiling. It was that very moment that the penny dropped – this was not a quick fix. This was serious.

What happened next?

Within only a few hours of being told my daughter has a life-long disease, I was giving her injections. I had never given anyone an injection before let along a 2-year old.

She was admitted and put on insulin immediately. Apparently we were lucky (?!) as with ketones of 4.6 she could have easily been unconscious or possibly in a coma. That was when the guilt came – why hadn't we noticed? Why did we not take her to the doctors sooner? What if she had gone unconscious?

Guilt then turned to anger – it wasn't fair. How can I do this? I know nothing about medication or caring in that capacity. It shouldn't be happening to me or my daughter. This sort of thing only happens to other families.

After that very sleepless night, I was left with fear and anxiety. Four years on and I still feel fear and anxiety for her but less frequently and over different things. We have learned to manage her diabetes, work through issues and give her the most 'normal' life as possible.

Over the next few days I was completely overwhelmed by the volume of information that I was expected to take in and remember. I panicked when Beatrice was discharged and we had to continue her care at home. We relied on her diabetes nurse for a tremendous amount of support.

We have now come to terms with Beatrice having type 1 diabetes and I can happily say that it does not dominate our lives anymore.

The disease does not define who my daughter is – my daughter is not *a* Type 1 Diabetic, instead she *has* Type 1 Diabetes. This may only be a small grammatical difference, but this difference is what enables Beatrice to live her life as other healthy children do.

Common comments made by others

If you have diabetes, you can't have sugar

Unfortunately there is still a significant lack of understanding of diabetes particularly the different types within it. More often than not, a persons' reaction to Beatrice is to not give her anything with sugar in. This is incredibly frustrating as it is not just sugar that is a problem, but carbohydrates (and now protein and fat in conjunction with carbohydrates) that can impact Beatrice's blood-glucose levels. There are times when Beatrice will need additional sugar for when she is hypoglycaemic and times when she will need more insulin to match her intake of carbohydrates. We cannot explain how important it is to us and to Beatrice that she is to have a varied diet which *will* include sugar and carbohydrates, the same as any other healthy child.

Your daughter has Type 1 diabetes because you have done something wrong as parents

This took a long time for me to accept as untrue and even now there are times when society's lack of understanding and assumptions can make me angry and blame myself in some way. You'll hear some people claim that diabetes is caused by a person being unfit or overweight or given too much sugar as a child. This is far from the truth. As a parent, it is your responsibility and your want to bring your child up happy and healthy. If they are not, you naturally feel it is your failing. It is not yet entirely understood as to why some people have type 1 diabetes over others but if it is caused by parental failings, than based on this environmental and nurture argument, our son should have it too. He does not. I once read on a social media site that type 1 diabetes is brought on by a stressful event in the person's life. There is no scientific evidence to prove that this is the case and I feel this may be a way for those affected to place blame and direct anger. I personally feel this is a destructive pathway and although some people may correlate having type 1 diabetes to a stressful event in their life, there are many people who have undergone stressful periods in their lives and not been diagnosed with type 1 diabetes. Rather than searching for a way to blame this disease on something or someone (and yes, far easier to say rather than do) as Bea's parents we felt it best to channel all our anger and frustration into understanding the disease and how best to manage it for her.

She'll grow out of it

No she won't! It's life long, but we will deal with it. There is on-going research into finding new and innovative ways of treating type 1 diabetes so the quality of Beatrice's life should only improve.

Coping with Type 1 diabetes as a toddler

The relentless hospital visits

Beatrice has had to learn to love the hospital and doctor's surgery. Rather than creating a place of urgency, stress and fear, we tried to make it an interesting place to visit. You would be amazed at how many toys that a paediatric hospital waiting room and ward have. All of which are apparently far better than the ones at home. Bea has become friends with the staff she routinely sees and makes games out of the blood pressure monitoring, finger pricking and tests done. The best part of having to visit hospital regularly from such a young age, is that whilst others her age would be put off by all the staff uniforms and equipment, they don't phase her one bit. In fact, she is quite fascinated by the mechanics of things and far braver than I could be. I have a photo of Bea's first admission when she was diagnosed. When I look at it I always smile – other than her little bandaged up arm covering her blood test ends in her hands, you'd have no idea she was in hospital. She is beaming due to the copious amounts of toys around her – the pretend vacuum cleaner was a hit. She is wearing a (clean!) urine sample bowl on her head and taking various people's temperature (?) with a stethoscope!

A toddlers interpretation of emotion

If your child is anything like Beatrice, then you'll know that getting any true assessment about how they are feeling is near impossible. Toddlers often say what they think their parent would like them to say as they want to please us. Although very endearing and thoughtful, this is quite problematic when it comes to determining whether they are out of the target blood-glucose range. There have been countless times when Bea is looking particularly peaky and on asking if she feels ok, it's always "oh yes, mummy I'm fine". Not entirely trusting this assessment of herself, I test her and more often than not the result is way below 4.0mmol. I was so worried that she would go through life claiming to be totally fine and then dropping unconscious on the floor. Yet you mustn't fret too much as once your child is at school age, their understanding of what feels 'normal' is far greater and their ability to communicate this develops and will continue to do so as they get older. Bea now gets that it is ok to admit that she feels "rubbish", it is not her fault and we won't be disappointed. There was a time when attempting to engage in a meaningful conversation (ridiculous with a toddler as really they just want to go and play) that I did find out that she felt that she disappointed us when she was 'low'. This was such a heart wrenching moment and yet again paved way for a whole new level of guilt. But in reality we forget how much these little sponges absorb. Inherently our children want to impress us and not let us down. Due to the stress and anxiety that a newly diagnosed child with diabetes can cause, a parent will inevitably demonstrate what appears to be disappointment on blood-glucose readings that are not within target range. As a parent we know that we are not disappointed with our child but instead are frustrated and possibly anxious or concerned with the reading (or disappointed with yourself – I'll come on to that later). Having friends who are parents of children without type 1 diabetes (I include parenting of my son in this too) that if it wasn't diabetes, your child would have these thoughts and feelings regardless but just about something else. Don't add this guilt to your probably already long list of worries you have. Just be aware that at the point you feel your child is able to understand (and sit still for more than 4 minutes without getting distracted) that it may be worth explaining that any reading outside target range is not their fault and we are not disappointed with them.

How type 1 diabetes affects behaviour

We have found that glucose levels running outside target range have a definite impact on Beatrice's behaviour. She can be moody, stubborn and adamantly claim the sun is green purely to have an argument for arguments sake. When Beatrice is exhibiting these behaviours at a heightened and irrational level, it is often a very good indicator that she is running high. When hypo, it soon became apparent that Beatrice will behave in one of two ways. She'll either be incredibly tired, pale and appear to be in a distant world; or she will be running around at speed, unable to follow any instructions being very silly as if high on adrenaline. In both situations when tested she will more often than not be in a state of hypoglycaemia.

Don't get me wrong, she can also exhibit these behaviours whilst in target range, but the key difference is that she is able to comprehend instruction and ultimately control her own behaviour unlike when she is hypo or hyper. When we talked to Beatrice about the difference in her behaviour, she explained that "when I'm normal and one side of my brain tells me to be naughty and silly and the other side tells me that I shouldn't I can listen to my good side but when I'm low or high I can't control my bad side." We often use these words to coax her down from her irrational behaviour when she is hyper and finding it difficult to communicate with her.

It is worth adding that despite managing glucose levels after a hyper, it can have a knock-on effect and quite often Beatrice's behaviour can be terrible for the remaining part of the day. I cannot give a scientific reason, but, most likely she is either overcome with tiredness that the hyper takes out of her, or there is still some residual adrenaline going round her.

As Beatrice is getting older, she is becoming more savvy and has been known to claim hyper or hypo excuses for her behaviour when in fact she is just being cheeky. We are able to call her bluff at times, but will test her blood regardless. We feel it is important to reinforce that she is not to use her having type 1 diabetes as an excuse for bad behaviour, particularly at school and when around those who do not have such a good understanding of the disease.

How Type 1 diabetes can impact your family

Wilfred, Beatrice's younger brother, was 9 months old when Beatrice was diagnosed. At that age Wilf was too young to have any idea that Beatrice was ill or have an understanding of her being any different from other big sisters. I can't tell you when Wilf realised Beatrice had diabetes but *I* remember the moment when *I* realised that he knew. I was due to take him to the doctors for a routine appointment one day. The morning of the appointment Wilfred was really agitated and was adamant he didn't need to go. I had no idea why he had got himself so upset so I plastered a smile on my face and wrestled him into his car seat. I was in the waiting room when Wilfie began sobbing and begged me not to stick needles in him. He said that he didn't want someone to take all his blood. Until this point it hadn't crossed my mind that Wilf felt fear in regards to Bea's diabetes. As far as he was concerned what Beatrice endured everyday was normal for every child and that he was to go through it too. The g-word filled me again and I realised, possibly a little late that we really should have talked to Wilfie about Bea's diabetes. I was so consumed in attempting to make Beatrice's life so 'normal' that we'd forgotten to have the same conversations with Wilfred. It took him a while to really understand that what Beatrice has is different from other children and he may or may not also have it at some stage but as this moment of his life, he doesn't. Ironically Beatrice has no fear of medicine, hospitals and openly talks about health and well-being, whereas Wilf has a strong fear of being ill and dislikes going to hospitals. I suppose he lives in fear that he may too be diagnosed with type 1 diabetes, despite our best efforts to reassure him. I write this not to alarm you, but to iterate that siblings only know what they are directly surrounded by unless told otherwise. If you have the opportunity it might be worth having some of the conversations with your child's siblings earlier than we did with Wilfred.

Wilfred is 4 years old now and in his first year of school. He understands that not all children have type 1 diabetes and has a good grasp on health, well-being and that Beatrice does have additional medicinal needs that he does not. As stated previously at this point in writing, there is no scientific evidence as to why some people have type 1 diabetes and others do not. As a family we decided to take part in a diabetes study to investigate this, with the knowledge that it will also give us the statistical probability of Wilfred being diagnosed with it. I can understand parents' concerns and decision not to have this information, however for us, we were happy to have this knowledge. We did have a scare last year that Wilfred had type 1 diabetes when he was frequently going to the toilet, drinking excessively and had a slightly higher than normal blood-glucose reading. Now being acutely aware of the symptoms, we whisked him to the doctors who then referred him to the hospital. They were very good but after 2 hours and blood-glucose reading being within the normal range, he was in fact diagnosed with a urine infection. Of course there is still a tiny bit at the back of my mind that there will always be chance Wilf could still have type 1 diabetes, but there is a chance that anyone could, so there is really is no point worrying about it now.

Living with type 1 diabetes affects other family members too. Both sets of Beatrice's grandparents live a little distance away from us so were never frequent babysitters due to logistics, however since Bea's diagnosis, we became aware of an unintentional resistance to looking after our children. At first I was frustrated but I now understand that it was fear that prevented them from looking after Beatrice. They were scared that they would get it wrong; they were scared that they would harm her in some way. They were overwhelmed by the volume of equipment and medicine that surrounds Bea's daily life. As Beatrice's primary carers we had little choice other than to deal with her diabetes and get on with it. By remembering the fear and anxiety I had when Bea was first diagnosed, I have now accepted the reaction of others. And it will not be too long before Beatrice becomes independent and self-sufficient in much of her diabetes that these fears will be reduced. If you are fortunate to have grandparents or childminders who are happy to take on the responsibility of a child with type 1 diabetes, ensure that you acknowledge their fears and concerns. Reflecting back on your own thoughts and feelings at diagnosis will help with this dialogue. And if you have family members who resist helping out, don't let their fears fuel resentment or allow become apparent to your child – they are not sophisticated enough to understand and will only feel that is somehow something they have done wrong.

The practicalities

I have talked mostly about emotions up until now, yet the practicalities and physical medical equipment that diabetes requires was an equal if not more of a concern for me. It is crazy how much stuff that you acquire in order to manage just the day to day affects of type 1 diabetes. My biggest piece of advice is to get organised! I admit that I am overly tidy and slightly obsessed with having no clutter in my house but I cannot stress the importance of being organised and tidy with all the equipment and medication that you'll have.

Storage – possibly something you will have already considered but if you use glucogels, injections or any other lotions remember to keep them somewhere that doesn't get overly hot or cold (we store all our kit in our downstairs WC shelf). I invested in a clever fishing tackle box as it has 2 layers and divided compartments for things. I fill each compartment with the lancets, batteries, ketone strips, testing strips, gels etc. And keep spare boxes of each in the bottom layer. Having the bits and pieces easily accessible and in one place makes life so much easier especially on a crazy school morning. We also dedicate one of the side shelves in our fridge for the opened insulin and emergency glucagon.

Of course if your child is using an insulin pump, then you'll have additional boxes of cartridges and cannulas to store. These come in quite large boxes and you'll likely order several boxes at a time so this will need a larger storage space. We keep ours in a large drawer upstairs out of the way of prying fingers.

Ordering – I won't lie, we must have visited the doctors about 4 times a week to renew prescriptions for the first few months as we were completely out of routine and kept forgetting what we would need and what would run out. Slowly we got ourselves together and now we have one complete repeat prescription list and we basically tick everything on it once every 2-3 weeks. There are times when more insulin or lancets may be required but generally our lovely prescription nurse doesn't have see me running in frantically asking for strips as we'd run out for the following day. With the pump we order 3 boxes of everything – don't forget your cartridge caps, battery caps and batteries! They are posted from abroad so will take a few days so again, you need to be a little forward thinking!

Kitchen scales – Do a bit of research, as these are crucial for accurate carb counting. I recommend those that don't require their own bowl or dish to measure in. Being able to use the plate or bowl that you dishing up on to is far easier. Electronic scales tend to be more accurate and try to get ones that have 'tare weight'. This is where the scales include a button which can reset the display to zero enabling see the different weight of each food as you add them to the scales. This is useful as each food will have different amounts of carbohydrates making it easier to carb count.

Notepad & pen – I carry one everywhere due to my list-making nature but always have pen & paper in the kitchen with the scales.

Calculator – keep it simple. A basic plastic one (no phone here - you'll inevitably splash food on it) will do the job but is essential to count carbs effectively.

Books – unless you really want to, reading manual after manual on diabetes is not essential to effective managing of your childs' diabetes. Attending the relevant courses, chatting to other parents (online forums can be useful, but again, don't get bogged down in things too early on) and having regular dialogues with your diabetes nurse is more than sufficient. However, I do recommend getting yourself a carb counting book for quick and easy carb counting on the go. It may be worth investing in a couple of these books as childminders and schools will benefit from having a copy (more on this later on).

Freebies – I only found this out about 3 months ago but check the brand of your blood-glucose meter as ours has a website that once you register your product you are able to order diaries, control solution and vouchers for replacement meter batteries all for free. This certainly saved us a few pounds.

Pump belts & pouches – there are several websites where you can purchase pump belts and cases. They are not cheap but rather than potentially destroying clothes (which they'll grow out of) or attempting to clip the pump the weight of small child's leg onto your little's one trousers which then end up around their ankles; I do recommend investing in a couple (trust me you'll need more than one as they'll get grubby!) They come in different width pouches and many are elasticated which proved best for Beatrice as she is so tiny.

Micro-managing – the pressure to get it right (all the time)

This section is mostly relevant to an insulin pump user due to the smaller units of insulin that can be given and the variety of settings that can be adjusted on the pump. However, elements of this are worth considering for those using injection pens when making changes to the daily insulin to carb ratios.

For me, trying to get good control of her diabetes is absolutely the most difficult aspect of Beatrice having the disease. I admit that I am the kind of person who takes pleasure in putting things in order and ensuring everything is neat, tidy and well organised. Naturally, I wanted Beatrice's levels to be perfect so coping with the unpredictably of type 1 diabetes was really difficult for me. My organised and logical mind could not cope with the number of variables that affect her levels. Foreseeing that she will spend time in a hot room as opposed to the lunch hall or anticipating that she will be in the sunshine more one day than another makes it impossible to micro-manage and control. I had to change my mindset and I realise now that it is more about the big picture with our focus now being to ensure that her levels are *generally* within target. For things that we are able to anticipate such as PE or a swimming lesson we make the relevant adjustments however, where previously I would have analysed each day's glucose readings tweaking everything, instead I now keep an eye on the readings but will only make changes when patterns occur, often making changes every few days. Obviously there are exceptions to this as if she running super high or low for the majority of the day, then clearly levels need to be altered a lot sooner.

Typically just when you think you have cracked it and have had a day or two of ideal target readings, suddenly things will spike up and down and all the settings will need changing. Most frustratingly though is when she is running high despite having increased both basals and bolus several times – almost doubling what she was having previously – and for her to continue to still run high. She'll be on target for a day and then suddenly all that insulin is no longer needed and she is hypo all the following day. Over the last couple of years we have noticed that this in itself is a pattern and ties in whenever she has a growth spurt or sudden change in routine e.g. first week back at school.

We found that getting into a routine helped us to manage Beatrice's levels. By allocating a convenient time once a week to upload all the data from the pump onto your computer, enabled us to have a conversation together and agree on the alterations for the week ahead. We found a Sunday morning a good time – often tying this in with battery and cap changes at the same time.

It is easy to blame yourself when you feel like you just can't the levels right but as I stated previously, there are so many variables that you cannot predict and so many possible changes you can make to the pump settings that sometimes it is overwhelming. At times when you feel like this is the case; it is time for you to contact your diabetes nurse. They are skilled in analysing glucose readings and more importantly, reassuring you that you are doing your best. Do not think that you should be doing this yourself – sometimes you just need a break from it and need an outsider to look at the big picture for you.

There are various ways to make adjustments to cope with spikes and dramatic changes, which I have discussed in the Pump Adjustments section.

Bed wetting

Beatrice wasn't quite at the stage of potty training at diagnosis but being her independent self, she wasn't far off. We bought a potty and got started with rewarding and giving her positive reinforcement whenever she communicated the need to go and made it to the potty on time. Happy days. We decided to leave it a while before nappy-free night times, thinking naively that this will be doddle. Of course those of you with older children will know that this is not the case. When you throw diabetes into the mix particularly at initial diagnosis where your child is likely to be running higher, it is even more of a challenge. Beatrice really struggled at night, with more bed-wetting nights than dry nights. Being honest as I feel I should, we did tell her off - many times – as we had not linked her bed wetting with diabetes. Changing bed sheets at 2am whilst half asleep does not bring out the most tolerant side of any parent. Don't underestimate the affect diabetes can have on the need to urinate. If your child is running high chances are that they are in such a deep sleep that they are not able to control the need to go. Quite often Beatrice would be completely unaware that she had wet the bed. We tried to limit her evening drinking but of course when hyper she would then wake up frequently in the night incredibly thirsty. Obviously we continued to adjust insulin levels but this in itself was another challenge (to be discussed later on). We then tried waking her up in the night to go but she would be so non-communicative that actually getting her into the bathroom was a nightmare. In the end, we stopped trying. She was dry during the day and we just popped on the pull-on sleep nappies at night. We realised that we were making this situation unnecessarily stressful for Beatrice and it wasn't actually bothering her that she wore nappies t night. When Bea started school (aged 5) we asked her what she wanted to do about night times (considering the possibility of sleepovers and school residential trips). This was 2 years after being nappy free during the day and 2.5 years after diagnosis. We were confident in how we were managing her diabetes so factoring in that she was more often within target range over night, as a family we thought we'd give it another try. Beatrice may not be great at getting out of bed at night but she is very good at alerting us of the need for her to go. Yes, it's a pain having to get out of bed at night to take her but it's far better – and saves on the washing – than her having an accident. Beatrice is now 6 years old and don't get me wrong, she still has accidents but with this open communication and with us having a greater understanding of the affects running hyper can have, she doesn't feel ashamed and we (try) not to show any frustrations at having to change her bed sheets. Essentially there is absolutely no point in rushing to be nappy-free at night, wait until you feel your child's diabetes is being controlled, then try. Trust me, getting frustrated and being knee deep in washing is not worth being dry a couple of nights a week for.

Dealing with hypos

At diagnosis the initial stage of managing your child's diabetes is about giving insulin to lower both ketones and glucose levels. Battling your child's hyperglycaemia is your main goal, and it is only later that you are aware of hypoglycaemia and the treating of hypos quickly and effectively is vital. There is no one size fits all treatment, as each person can respond differently to different sugars. We find the energy tablets and gels work best for Beatrice as they are the fastest at bringing her levels up to target range. Other people swear by jelly babies, energy drinks, fizzy drink or even chocolate bars. Unfortunately treating hypos can be costly as other than the glucogels there is no free treatment available on the NHS.

Initially knowing how much sugar your child needs to combat a hypo is guess work. Over time it will become instinctual in knowing how much to give your child. Beatrice is at a point now that she is very good at telling us what she thinks she might need.

Of course, treating a hypo is not always this easy. It is typically the middle of the night when Beatrice has a severe hypo. I class a severe hypo (this is not a medical definition) as one that spans over more than an hour and where her blood glucose levels continues to fall as opposed to going up to target range despite being given sugar. On nights like this, we can get through several tubes of gel, countless tablets and resorting to biscuits and anything else that she is able to consume. At the point of writing we have been lucky in that despite being as low as 1.7mmol Beatrice has never lost consciousness or passed out. This has enabled us to get food into her but for those who do pass out, having gels to hand is important as they can be ingested by rubbing into their cheek rather than having to actively swallow. Your diabetes nurse may also have given you a prescription for a glucagon injection. This is a very quick and effective way of administering glucose into the human body and generally only used for severe hypos. It is not expected that you administer it yourself as a paramedic will carry one with them, however it is good to be familiar with how to administer the glucagon as it is different from an injection pen. We have not yet had to use the glucagon on Beatrice.

The first few times that Beatrice experienced severe hypos I contacted the diabetes centre at hospital for support. I found that they will trust your parental instincts but will always offer for you to bring your child in if you have any concerns. Don't be afraid to ring as often as you feel you need to – this is what the diabetes team are there for. Equally, if you are very concerned then do not hesitate to call an ambulance. We have had only needed to call out the emergency services once ourselves, and the paramedic stayed until he was confident that Beatrice was back in range and we were happy to take over. Throughout her time at pre-school an ambulance was called out twice due to severe hypos, and again although the glucagon injection was not needed, the paramedics stayed with a back up ambulance on call until everyone felt confident that Beatrice would be ok. A severe hypo is not necessarily a result of poorly managed diabetes or bad parenting. They happen to even the most perfectly micro-managed people with type 1 diabetes and you will not be judged on it.

A related concern to treating hypos was the affect the additional sugar, particularly during the night, was having on Beatrice's teeth. I spoke to the dentist about it and in addition to the obvious brushing of her teeth twice a day, they were able to put extra fluoride onto her teeth. It may not always be necessary but it is worth mentioning if you feel your child's teeth are becoming affected.

Being ill with type 1 diabetes

If it isn't bad enough having a small child with sickness and diarrhoea, you haven't experienced a child with type 1 diabetes with it. It puts a whole new spin on things...

Firstly all that insulin you gave your child to balance the foods that they have eaten – well that insulin is still in their body nicely bringing down their blood-glucose except that they no longer have this food in them. So, this will trigger a hypo. So after being sick you now have to try and get them to eat a dry powdery glucose tablet, a gunky gel or some sort of sugary sweet. Not particularly appealing for them. Oh and you'll be thinking of your usual trick of suspending the insulin pump or not give them an injection until their blood-glucose is back in target. But no – you can't because their ketones will be high – and I mean they could go super high. This is dangerous. So you have to go through the nightmare balancing act of giving them more insulin to combat the ketones whilst attempting to feed your toddler even more sugar food to ensure they don't hypo further. And to top it off, I guarantee it'll be in the middle of the night when your amazing diabetes nurse is off-duty and you only have the out-of-hours hospital phone number. And by morning your lovely child will be sleeping peacefully while you feel like you have gone through world war 3. We've gone through this countless times and Beatrice is fine. But that first time – it is scary and seriously confusing, which is why you must make the most of the help available to you. Contact your diabetes nurse first, they'll talk things through with you on the phone, or contact the paediatric diabetes ward at hospital. If you are really struggling or you really can't get your child back to normal ketones or out of hypo, take them in to hospital. I remember Beatrice being ill all night and it got to the point where dad had to sleep on the floor in her bedroom as she was lacking so much energy she couldn't make it to the bowl let alone the toilet!

You'll be fine, just stay calm and follow the sick day rules that your diabetes nurse gives you. My golden rule – don't underestimate the importance of checking ketones. Get them right and then sort out hypos.

Moving from injections to the pump

I didn't want Beatrice to move onto the pump. I had so many 'what if...' questions that I had convinced myself that the pump was an awful bit of machinery that would ruin my precious little girl's life. In reality I was terrified at what it represented. In my mind, having type 1 diabetes already made her different to all the other children and having a pump would be a visual reminder that she was going to be permanently different to others.

I needed a lot of convincing that having an insulin pump would actually enable Beatrice to lead a more 'normal' life. This was one of the lower points for me as a parent with a newly diagnosed child with type 1 diabetes and I became a little withdrawn. My husband did some research and showed me pictures of sporting heroes that also had type 1 diabetes. I'm not big into sport but seeing images of fit and healthy adults who were achieving great things due to the benefits of the pump did hit home. I realised Beatrice would be incredibly lucky to have this piece of equipment to act as her pancreas and it would enable her to live her life without type 1 diabetes dictating what she can and can't do.

Don't get me wrong I still had a lot of questions and concerns:

Won't the tubing get tangled?

The tubes are pretty invincible as they are bendy and flexible and have an outer tubing to protect the inner tube carrying the insulin. Beatrice has been using a pump for over 3 years now and has never broken or split the tubing. She even went through a stage of chewing the tubing for comfort when she was bored, and although the outer tubing looked damaged, the insulin was still protected inside.

It is very difficult to tangle or get knots in, the worst that happens is when she gets it wrapped round herself before and after the toilet but it doesn't do any damage.

Will it hurt her?

Generally no, it does not hurt when you insert the cannula into Beatrice's body. To have an understanding of how it feels, I have inserted an empty and unattached cannula into my own body. I left it in for a couple of days similarly to how Beatrice would leave hers and after 5 minutes I had very little awareness that it was there. Beatrice was only 2 and half when she got her pump so had very little fat on her which meant that we were limited in the number of injection sites we could use. We rotated around her tummy so that it would not get in the way of her nappy and as she got older we rotated the injection sites to include her bottom. Surprisingly having the cannula on her bottom cheeks is not uncomfortable when she sits down, contrary to what we had expected. There are also a variety of barrier lotions that can be used if you find the cannulas aren't sticking to your child's skin or leave red sore marks when you remove them.

Of course there will be occasions that the cannula needle hits muscle especially when Beatrice is tensing in anticipation. It can be a little painful but will last no longer than a few seconds.

It is important that the sites are rotated at each cannula change to reduce the risk of little bumps forming on their bodies. Your diabetes nurse should examine your childs injection sites at clinic appointments and check for these lumps. Do not worry too much though as you can only do your best on a limited amount of body space and remember that children grow so fast that the injection areas will expand. Using her bottom as a primary injection site was to help hides any lumps that may form.

Won't it get in the way when playing sport?

There are various ways in which the pump can be carried with your child. The pump comes with a clip on the back which can be used to attach it onto clothes. You can slip the pump into pockets or invest in a couple of neoprene/lycra belts that the pump sits in and can be worn under or over clothes (see pump belts & pouches in the Practicalities section). Beatrice has gone through nursery, pre-school and primary school wearing her pump as well as doing PE lessons, swimming lessons, bike rides, ballet and typical children's' play in the park and garden. Never has she said that the pump has got in the way or prevented her taking part in these activities.

Of course, if you are really concerned that it will get in the way during a particular activity, the pump can be temporarily disconnected from your child. Ensure that the pump is suspended and then resumed for no longer than two hours, remembering to test your child blood levels during the activity. There has only been one occasion that we disconnected Bea from her pump (other than the weekly data upload) and that was on a trip to the beach with rather frantic sea splashing combined with hot sun made us decide to remove the pump for an hour.

What about bath time or swimming?

The pump is waterproof so can be worn in water. However, to reiterate from earlier, I would strongly recommend that you routinely check your pump over for cracks and scratches and regularly change the battery and cartridge caps to keep the pump in peak condition. Depending on how your child's blood glucose levels are affected by activity in a warm swimming pool area you may decide to disconnect the pump as typically Beatrice does not require constant insulin during a swimming session so often it makes sense to remove the pump.

What if it stops working?

The pump will be attached to your child for 24 hours a day 7 days a week therefore it is inevitable that it will stop working at some point in their life time. It has happened twice with Beatrice through no fault of our own. When your pump stops working you will need to revert back to injections until you receive a working pump. The key to coping when this happens is to frequently upload data from your pump to your online data centre where you can view all your pumps settings from the latest upload. You can use these to work out the insulin to carb ratio and the daily basal total which can be given via injection. On both occasions that Beatrice needed a replacement pump, it was a really quick and easy process. They sent out a new pump the next working day with a box for you to return the broken one.

To keep the pump performing as it should, get into a routine of changing the battery and cartridge caps as they can get surprisingly mucky. At each upload we give the pump a quick check looking for any cracks and scratches. If you spot any cracks, contact your pump supplier immediately.

There will be days that your child's blood glucose readings may be different to what you expect. This could be due to many reasons but if your child is running very high despite being given corrections, it is worth changing the cannula as often the short bit of tube can go into the injection site at an angle and bend, therefore not giving the correct dose of insulin. This has only happened a handle of times in the 3 and half years that Beatrice has been on the pump.

Insurance

Your child's pump is an expensive bit of equipment and is a substitute pancreas for them. Your pump supplier will replace a faulty pump but will not replace one that has been lost, stolen or accidently damaged so it is essential that you get it insured. Check the level of cover available on your house insurance as some companies will not cover items for accidental damage or when they are removed from the house. We have listed Beatrice's pump as a specified personal item for the value of what it would cost to replace it. In addition we have specified a second diabetes pump to cover us for when we take a spare pump on holiday.

It's too complicated!

Before you are let loose on an insulin filled pump you will be given a vial of saline for you to practice with. It will allow you to be familiar in changing cannulas and administering medication using the different options on the pump.

It will be a steep learning curve in becoming familiar with the various settings on the pump but rest assured that you will not be alone and are not expected to make any changes on your own until you are ready. You diabetes nurse will set up the pump's initial settings for you and will contact you every few days to check how things are going and make any adjustments that are needed.

I remember our first cannula change and having all the bits laid out on the table along with the instruction booklet. I was so paranoid I'd do it wrong that it took me at least 20 minutes and three cartridge and cannula kits later to just about got it right. Now, it takes no more than 30 seconds whilst Bea gets dressed in the mornings.

It is a gradual process and you will feel anxious. I worried that the cannula wasn't inserted properly or I'd given Beatrice insulin for carbs instead of a correction for a blood glucose level and then I'd forget if I'd primed the cannula first but as long as you keep doing blood glucose tests, it can all be managed.

How will others know how to use it?

It's about confidence and control. Both myself and Adrian are confident in how we manage Beatrice's diabetes and although we strive for her blood glucose levels to be in target we know that it will never be perfect, or at least, not perfect for very long. Mistakes will be made and blood glucose levels will be irregular. Allowing someone else to care for Beatrice for the first time was very hard. We had to put all faith into Beatrice's pre-school teachers who'd never used a pump before and trust that they would give the correct amount of insulin at the right time in the right way. Although I was worried, it was important for us not to transfer how nervous we were to her teachers as it would only make them feel less confident.

We want people to feel confident in caring for Beatrice and not to worry if they make a mistake. Mistakes have only happened twice since Beatrice has been on the pump and both times her teacher phoned me immediately. The teacher had forgotten to put the carbs that Beatrice had eaten at lunchtime into her pump. The problem was solved quickly and Beatrice was absolutely fine. Later, the teacher said that as we were so calm and didn't make her feel worse than she already felt, she consequently felt more confident in using the pump as we'd removed her anxiety in making mistakes. Don't get me wrong, I can appear calm and laid back on the outside when in fact I'm actually frantically panicking on the inside to come up with a solution.

In practical terms, the simplest way to ensure that others caring for your child know what they are doing is to not give them too much information. They are unlikely to need to know how to alter any of the settings on the pump. Instead, they will need to know only how to enter any carbohydrates eaten and how to enter a blood glucose reading with or without a correction. These instructions can be written down – I have two laminated sets that I've made and just hand over whenever someone looks after her.

What if she fiddles with the pump and accidently gives herself insulin?

Beatrice has done this on several occasions, most often at night when she is in bed and has nothing else to do other than fiddling with her pump. Like most children she isn't daft and worked out how to unlock her pump pretty early on. Routinely, you will frequently test her blood so no more than an hour had past when we tested her next in the evening and found her running hypo. Not sure why she had an unexpected low we checked the pump history (amazing tool!) and found she had given herself 2 units of insulin. Obviously this is dangerous and could have ended in a much worse situation but it didn't and instead we needed to come up with a method of prevention. In the morning we had a stern conversation with her but at two years old, this wasn't going to be much of a deterrent. We decided to put the pump in a zippy pouch and padlocked the zips together so she couldn't take it out. It sounds dramatic but I had to be realistic in the potential danger that Beatrice having access to pump could cause. Beatrice is 6 years old now and I believe it has been 18 months since we felt the need to padlock her pump to her. She now has a good understanding that it's not a toy and that her pump saves her life but could also seriously harm her if she does not use it correctly.

Pump Adjustments

There are a number of settings that can be adjusted on the pump. Your diabetes nurse will go through them with you and advise you on what alterations to make. This will be in addition to the pump manual that explains in detail how to use your pump.

I have put together a basic list of the primary options and settings that you are likely to use in the initial stages of pump use, although does depend on the brand of pump that your child will use.

- Basal

This is the background insulin that is constantly being administered over 24 hour periods. The amounts of insulin are set using blocks of time and can be adjusted depending on how much is required at different times of the day.

- Bolus

This is insulin that you administer either when your child has eaten carbohydrates or when entering a blood glucose reading into the pump as a correction dose. The ratios of insulin to carbohydrates can be set using different time blocks.

- Normal Bolus

This is the most basic way of giving insulin but often rarely used. This is when you want to give additional insulin above a correction dose such as when you need to give extra insulin to bring down high ketones. You can choose the number of units of insulin to give at the point of entry rather than based on pre-set ratios or time intervals.

- BG

After doing a finger prick test using the blood/glucose meter, the reading is entered into the pump via a BG setting. Quite simply it logs the data and will administer a correction dose if required.

- Carbs

When carb counting, the number of carbohydrates eaten is entered into the pump. The pump will then give the pre-set amount of insulin depending on number of carbs entered.

- Combo Bolus

You are unlikely to use the combo bolus option until you are a confident pump user as it is a more complex way of administering insulin. However, once you have got to grips with it, it is incredibly useful for high GI foods that release carbohydrates slowly such as pasta; or when eating a combination of carbohydrates and protein such as pizza. It works by allowing you to specify how much insulin to give over a certain amount of time unlike the previous methods which give all the insulin in one go.

For example, if Beatrice has pasta totalling 80g of carbohydrates, rather than giving her all 80g carbohydrates at once, we spread the insulin over a selected amount of time. There is no blanket ratio as it can differ for everyone but after plenty of trial and error we have found that a ratio of 40:60% over 2 hours works well with Beatrice. This means that 40% of the insulin is given immediately and the remaining 60% is spread over a 2 hour time frame.

The combo bolus is also useful when Beatrice is grazing as you can spread the total amount of insulin over a set amount of time. The most common use of the combo bolus for us is when Beatrice goes to a birthday party or a friend's house for tea. We can enter the number of carbohydrates into the pump when we drop her off using a ratio of 0:100% over a one hour time span. This sets the pump to give all the insulin for the number of carbohydrates we predict that Beatrice will eat over one hour. This is much easier than trying to explain how to use the pump to someone who is unlikely to use it often.

- I:C ratio

The I:C ratio is the ratio of insulin to carbohydrates consumed. It is important to change this ratio for different time blocks as your child will require different amounts of insulin for the carbohydrates eaten at different points during the day. By doing regular uploads of data you can view several days' worth of pump data which will help in identifying a pattern of high or low glucose readings. Again, there is no set rule and you won't always get it right first time, but by getting into habit of tweaking settings you are on track to well-managed diabetes.

It is typical that just as we think we have got the ratios right for Beatrice, she'll have a growth spurt or her school routine will change and we will need to adjust the ratio again. Over time you will notice patterns, for example Beatrice has a lot more insulin for carbohydrates at breakfast whereas later in the day she'll need much less.

- ISF ratio

The Insulin Sensitivity Factor ratio is how the correction dose of insulin is programmed into the pump. Although you are unlikely to make your own adjustments to this, it is useful to be aware of this setting so you can make the suggested alterations as advised by your diabetes nurse at clinic appointments.

School, child-minding and babysitting

When Beatrice was initially diagnosed with type 1 diabetes to say I was reluctant to let anyone babysit her is an understatement. I was overwhelmed with information and equipment even with the diabetes training, so there was no way I was happy to let anyone else look after her. However, long term, this was unrealistic and once Beatrice returned to pre-school I realised that it wouldn't be too long before we had to let someone babysit her.

The key was to let those caring for Beatrice to take as much control as they were willing. I want them to feel confident in making decisions, whether this is to decide to give her a biscuit before PE because she is in a low target zone, or to give her only half the insulin as they predict she will only eat half her meal. The more I am checking up on them, the less confident they will feel in looking after Beatrice and more likely to make mistakes.

I remember Beatrice's first day at school – I don't think I slept the previous night due to nerves and anxiety. What if they forget to test her? What if she is hypo and her teacher hasn't noticed? What if they don't count the carbohydrates correctly? The reality is that in the short time between blood/glucose tests it is highly unlikely that anything that terrible would happen to Beatrice and that whoever is caring or Beatrice are just as worried about making mistakes as I am.

It must have been a week into Beatrice's first term at school when her class teacher called me in panic. She was worried that she'd done something awful. Of course I was silently panicking until she said "I tested her at 2.20pm instead of 2pm, I'm so sorry, I totally forgot. We've been testing her all afternoon since as we were so worried that we'd harmed her." I had to reassure her that it really was ok and would not dramatically affect Beatrice. Since then Beatrice's teacher relaxed and began making decisions without phoning me first. Later into the term, when discussing Beatrice and how well the school were managing her diabetes, the teacher said that the reason she felt she could take control was purely down to my reaction to that first mistake she had made. By (appearing) laid back and accepting the mistake she felt reassured and more confident to care for Beatrice.

In practical terms, the best way for good diabetes control between carers is open communication. We keep a diabetes diary that we log her levels and targets in and hand it to the school staff in the mornings to record blood glucose levels, number of carbs eaten and how they treat any hypos. We encourage them to contact us if they were ever unsure of what they are doing and to contact the hospital or ambulance if they feel the need.

I produced a simple set of instructions which I gave the school and put together an 'emergency' supply box of infusion kits, tablets, gels, batteries and lancets.

Take it a step at a time with babysitters, by timing it after your child has had tea and are in bed (and given the overnight insulin if on injection pens), a babysitter will only be required to do a blood/glucose test and treat a hypo if necessary. Only give them the information that they need to know – they don't need to be able to count carbs or know how to make changes and adjustments to the pump or inject insulin. You are only a phone call away and a phone call to the diabetes team or ambulance is an option if your babysitter is very concerned.

Uniform

This is not a massive issue but one worth mentioning as it is not so easy to customise school uniform and some schools may have a strict uniform policy.

When Beatrice was very little she was too slight to cope with the pump being clipped onto her trouser or skirt waistbands as it would pull her clothes down. So we opted for a pump belt which went over her trousers or underneath her skirt as she wanted it hidden. We continued with this when she started school not realising that it meant that the school staff would be required to lift Beatrice's skirt to get to the pump. This of course put them in a compromising position so we changed to putting the belt over the top of her skirt and threading the tubing underneath and up and over the skirt waistband.

As Beatrice has grown, her preference is to use the pump clip to attach the pump to the waistband of her school skirts. In summer, we chose a buttoned summer dress with pockets so she can thread the pump tube through a gap between buttons and then slip it into her pocket rather than using a pump belt.

For boys, they will likely have multiple pockets in their school shorts and trousers so can clip the pump onto the waistband or slip into their pocket. They may still prefer a pump belt as it will keep the pump more secure whilst they run around rather than bouncing around in a pocket.

PE

Beatrice's first term at school didn't go as smoothly as I had anticipated as we didn't have a great handle on days when she had PE.

Problem 1 - After the painstaking mission of getting plimsolls that didn't fall of her feet and a PE t-shirt that would have adequate growing room, we had completely forgotten to consider where her pump would attach to her PE kit. I think her first couple of PE lessons involved some weird and wonderful belts made out of the teacher's scarves and inventive methods of clipping the pump to her so it wouldn't fall off whilst she is running around. So although your child's teacher may be equally as inventive, make sure you remember to pack a spare a pump belt or clip in your child's PE kit bag.

Problem 2 – Bea frequently hypo'd after PE. Regardless as to whether your child is using injections or a pump, it is really important that your child's blood/glucose is tested before and after PE. Even when Bea's reading was above 4.0mmol before PE she would often hypo afterwards. For pump users you are likely to have the same basal intervals for each day so your pump will not take into account the additional exercise on certain school days. After plenty of trial and error we have counter-acted this by deciding that if Beatrice's blood/glucose reading is below 6.0mmol before PE then she is to be given an 11g carb biscuit before hand with the carbohydrates for the biscuit not being put into the pump. This has helped in keeping Beatrice in range during and after PE. This is not a one-size-fits-all approach but it is worth keeping snacks at school for those PE days if you find that your child's blood/glucose readings are affected by PE.

Problem 3 – The weather. As above, the additional exercise that PE involves affects Beatrice's levels, but where she takes part in PE also makes a difference. During the summer when the days are hot, her levels are likely to run lower due to the heat. So, when she doing PE outside on a hot day, she will likely run even lower. Therefore, we might adjust her basal rate in the morning of her PE day to give her less insulin to account for this, or she may require additional carbohydrates in the form of a snack beforehand.

Carbohydrate counting and eating out

Always have a calculator and a pen and paper with you, particularly at the beginning where you are still learning which foods are carbohydrates and needing to calculate carbohydrates per weight.

There are a number of ways of tackling carb counting when out and about:

Ask for a copy of the nutritional information – nearly all chain restaurants or fast food places have printed lists of nutritional content per food item.

Check out their websites/app – Some places have the nutritional information on their website or app so if you know you will be eating out somewhere you can plan ahead and bring the information with you. This will also help when giving insulin before food as you can anticipate the number of carbohydrates to give before the food arrives.

Bring scales – don't be afraid to bring a set of scales with you if you want to. I know for the first few weeks I carried a set in the car as I wanted the carb counting to be as accurate as possible. If anyone questions you, it is good opportunity to educate them on the difficulties that type 1 diabetes can bring.

Look at the packaging – nearly everything has the nutritional content written on the packaging. Do however be mindful that you are using the correct values for what you are calculating – most products display both the carbohydrates in 100g weights and in portion sizes.

Carb counting book or app – we have several copies of a carb counting book. There are alternative books available but I recommend choosing one that has pictures of the food in various sized portions on plates so you can easily compare what is on your childs plate to the pictures in the book or on the app. Some of the books have full meals in them too to help when you have several carbohydrates on the plate.

Make a list of frequently eaten foods – I have a written list of foods that Beatrice commonly eats with their corresponding carbohydrate content for quick reference. I also cut out the nutritional information lists off some packaging that I would normally discard after purchase e.g. yogurt pot cardboard and keep together so I don't have to rummage through recycling a few days later to find (yes, I've done it).

Subscribe to a food magazine – many food magazines have the nutritional values printed at the end of recipes. These are great as it means you don't need to worry about calculating each ingredient individually. Just make sure you read the number of servings that the recipe is written for and then divide up the carbohydrates accordingly. You may find you initially lean towards magazines targeted at those with food related illnesses and these are useful but most food magazines are equally as good, and can have a wider variety of recipes which you can feed the whole family rather than design meals specifically for your child with type 1.

Calculating carbohydrates

You may feel overwhelmed at the beginning and even just identifying which foods are carbohydrates will feel a challenge let alone calculating the number of carbohydrates per portion. It does get easier and you will surprise yourself in how quickly you remember the carbohydrate content in commonly eaten foods just by the frequent carb counting.

A reminder of calculating carbohydrate content:

$$\frac{Amount\ of\ carbs\ in\ 100g\ of\ food}{100} \times weight\ of\ food\ on\ plate$$

So, if there are 30g carbs per 100g of food, and there is 25g of the food on your child's plate, calculate the total number of carbs to be eaten by:

$$\frac{30}{100} \times 25$$

If the nutritional information states that there 26g per 85g of food and your child has 34g of the food, the total carbohydrates consumed would be:

$$\frac{26}{85} \times 34 = 10.4g\ carbs\ consumed$$

'Diabetic' chocolate and sweets

I really dislike foods that you see in shops claiming to be for diabetics. Firstly, I don't like the label 'diabetics', Beatrice isn't the illness, she's not diabetic; she has the illness, therefore has diabetes. Secondly, they really don't taste very nice and the reason that they claim to be for people with diabetes is because the manufacturer has omitted the sugar content. In order for the product to still taste sweet they have replaced the sugar with artificial sweeteners, which is my third reason for disliking them. They are over-priced chocolate which taste awful and are filled with numerous other artificial ingredients that are not going to be any healthier for a child. Beatrice will eat the usual chocolate or sweets that Wilfred has and I count the carbs for it instead.

Travelling with type 1diabetes

My rule is to plan for the worst i.e. constant hypos, sickness requiring additional insulin and loss of injection pens or test kits... It does mean that you will pretty much end up bringing an entire additional suitcase with you, but this is still a lot easier that having to track down a pharmacy or doctor who is able to understand what you require and actually get for you fast enough. I recommend bringing the following:

- Blood/glucose meter and finger pricker
- Spare blood/glucose meter and finger pricker
- Ketone test meter
- Both injection pens
- Fresh full vials of insulin for injection pens
- Additional insulin vial for the pump
- Spare pump
  - Contact your pump provider before you travel to order a spare pump to take with you. They will need advance notice so do not leave this to the last minute. They will send you a spare pump which you return to them on return from your travels.
- A very recent upload of data from the pump
- Printed list of settings from the pump
  - This is accessible from the pump's data centre. You should take a copy of the pump's settings including amount of basal insulin given over 24 hours and insulin to carb ratios. This is so you are prepared should you need to revert to injections whilst away.
- Spare batteries and caps for the pump
- Spare batteries for the blood/glucose meter
- Spare box of lancets
- Several boxes of test strips
- Several boxes of ketone test strips
- Several boxes of glucose gels
- Several tubs of fast acting glucose tablets

- Cannulas, inset cartridges and infusion kits for pump
    - Bring more than you think you'll need as your child is likely to be more active whilst on holiday so there is a higher risk of cannulas getting knocked about and if on a beach holiday, you may want to change cannulas more frequently if concerned about sand getting in them.
- Scales
- Calculator
- Letter from your GP or diabetes nurse
    - This covers you for having to travel with medication and equipment when going through luggage control.
- List of all the prescriptions
    - In case you do run out of supplies, having a list of prescriptions will make it a lot easier to get what you need
- Adequate insurance
    - You should already have the insulin pump included on your house insurance, but check as many companies may not covers the pump when abroad as standard. In addition, whichever travel insurance you go with, ensure that your child's type 1 diabetes is specifically identified as an illness on the policy.
- Sharps bin
    - We take a little sharps bin with us so we can dispose of needles responsibly.
- Storing all the kit
    - We keep all the above kit in a separate holdall from the rest of our luggage and make it the last bag we pack into the car so it is easy to get to. When transporting any unopened insulin it should be kept cold. There are various special insulin storage boxes available to buy online so it is worth having a shop around for what would be suitable for your needs.

Monetary support

The likelihood is that you will have already been informed by your diabetes nurse that your child is eligible for some monetary support in the form of Disability Living Allowance (DLA). The money can be paid in monthly instalments directly into your bank account and can be a substantial amount. Although you may feel this is not your priority and may feel guilty with idea of receiving money for your child's illness, please don't! No one actually thinks you are happy to have a child with type 1 diabetes just so you can receive benefits. As you may have already discovered, caring for a child with type 1 is hard work! You will be up during the night treating never-ending hypos, you will be called away from work and traipsing to the pharmacy, doctors, hospital, clinic appointments regularly and you will spend money on sweets, glucose tablets, drinks etc. You deserve the money, it helps, and put it towards whatever you choose. Some parents use it to help finance the CTG sensors that are currently not on the NHS, whereas some put it towards general living expenses, others save it for an annual holiday. The bottom line is though; please ensure you receive the monetary support that you deserve.

The next steps

Beatrice will continue to have good days and bad days. I don't doubt that she'll rebel against her diabetes as a teenager but I can say with certainty that she will not let type 1 diabetes define her. I know that she will use diabetes as an excuse for things, and why shouldn't she? Beatrice knows when take to take diabetes seriously but realistically if it wasn't diabetes, she'd play me in a different way! It makes me happy when she is acknowledging her diabetes in a positive way. It will be part of her forever, it can't be ignored, shamed or viewed negatively.

She's a strong willed, independent and sporty individual. As her mum, I know I will continue to worry about her but I will also continue to worry about her brother who doesn't have type 1 diabetes - it is just part and parcel of being a parent.

I am optimistic for the future as treatment for type 1 diabetes has progressed massively and will continue to do so with the amount of on-going research and trials being conducted.

Acknowledgements

Writing this has been far more emotional than I was expecting it to be and has brought me to tears numerous times. It has been a therapeutic experience being able to admit my thoughts and feelings to paper using my experience to hopefully help others.

I have mentioned very little of my husband, Adrian, in this book but this bears no reflection on the amount he has contributed in the care and support of our daughter, Beatrice. He has been the person I can be utterly honest with in regards to the guilt, frustration, fear and anger I had and still have with type 1 diabetes. Equally, he is by my side when caring for Bea's hypos, melt downs and midnight sickness. It was Adrian who stayed by Beatrice's side throughout her admission to hospital at diagnosis stage. I cannot thank him enough for carrying our family through what felt at times like crisis.

Wilfred is the best younger brother that Beatrice could have. He is calm, kind and caring. A real ying to her yang. He has had to be so patient and cope with being second many times when Beatrice's diabetes has been priority. He may only be 4 years old but he has never complained. I know he will always look out for her.

Beatrice's grandparents have to be mentioned as they have taken on the responsibility of all the paraphernalia that goes along with caring for Beatrice. It was a steep learning curve for them and I must thank them for enabling Adrian and I to have some much needed time out.

Thank you also to the wonderful diabetes team at Treliske Hospital for all their hard work, support, smiles and positive attitudes. We would never have coped so well without all the support available to us from them. They truly are a wonderful bunch of people.

Beatrice's first day at school was such an anxious time for me, but Portreath School have been wonderful. A great set of teachers and teaching assistants who have all treated Beatrice as though she is their own. They have given me confidence in allowing Beatrice to be independent and have faith that she will be fine without me by her side.